THE DASH DIET COOKBOOK FOR HYPERTENSION

Easy, Healthy Recipes to Lower Blood Pressure and Prevent Hearth Stroke.

Emma Fox

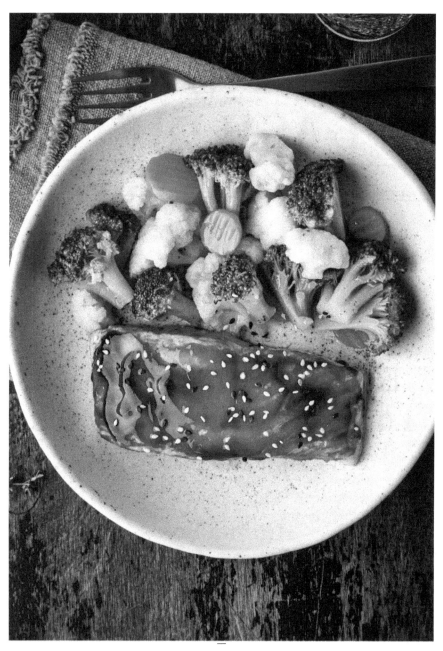

The information in the following pages is broadly considered a truthful and accurate account of facts and as such, any inattention, use, or misuse of the information in question by the reader will render any resulting actions solely under their purview. There are no scenarios in which the publisher or the original author of this work can be in any fashion deemed liable for any hardship or damages that may befall them after undertaking information described herein.

Additionally, the information in the following pages is intended only for informational purposes and should thus be thought of as universal. As befitting its nature, it is presented without assurance regarding its prolonged validity or interim quality. Trademarks that are mentioned are done without written consent and can in no way be considered an endorsement from the trademark holder.

TABLE OF CONTENTS

BREAKFAST

Banana-Berry Smoothie

Ready in about: 10 min
Serves: 1
Per serving:
Kcal 180, Sodium 95 mg, Protein 8 g, Carbs 33 g, Fat 2 g

INGREDIENTS:
- ½ ripe banana, preferably frozen
- ½ cup fresh or frozen blueberries
- ½ cup low-fat (1/%) milk
- ½ cup plain low-fat yogurt
- ¼ tsp. vanilla extract
- 1 tbsp. amber agave nectar (optional)

DIRECTIONS:

Peel and cut the banana into pieces. Combine all ingredients, including sweetener (if using), in a blender until smooth. Transfer into a tall glass and serve immediately.

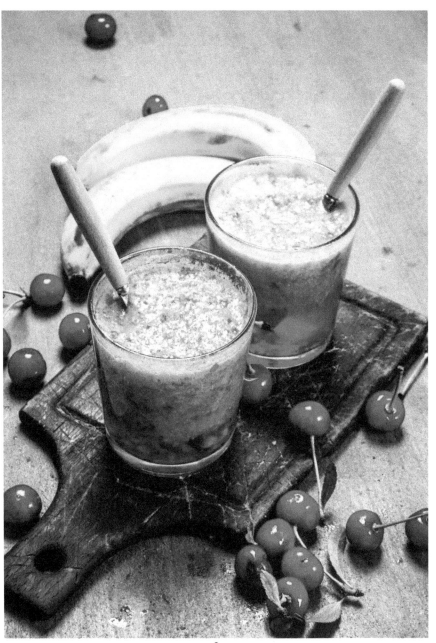

Berries Deluxe Oatmeal

Ready in about: 20 min
Serves: 2
Per serving:
Kcal 261, Sodium 115 mg, Protein 7 g, Carbs 63 g, Fat 10 g

INGREDIENTS:

- 1½ cups unsweetened plain almond milk
- ⅛ tsp. vanilla extract
- 1 cup old-fashioned oats
- ¾ cup mix of blueberries, blackberries, and coarsely chopped
- strawberries
- 2 tbsp. toasted pecans

DIRECTIONS:

Heat the vanilla and almond milk in a saucepan over medium heat. The moment the mixture starts to simmer, add the oatmeal and stir for about 4 minutes, or until most of the liquid is absorbed. Add the berries. Pour the mixture into two bowls and garnish with a toasted pecan.

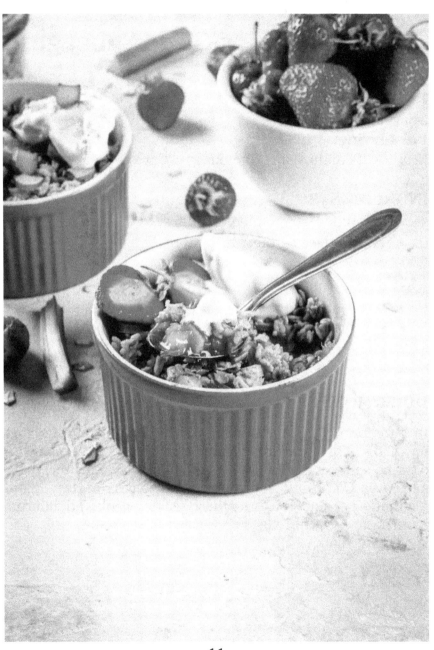

Lean Country-Style Sausage

Ready in about: 15 min
Serves: 6
Per serving:
Kcal 109, Sodium 52 mg, Protein 15 g, Carbs 1 g, Fat 4 g

INGREDIENTS:
- ½ pound lean ground pork loin
- ½ pound lean ground turkey breast
- 1 tsp. sugar
- 1 tsp. dry mustard
- 1 tsp. onion powder
- 1 tsp. sage
- 1 tsp. ground black pepper
- ½ tsp. red pepper flakes (optional)

DIRECTIONS:

In an enormous bowl, combine all the ingredients. Form 12 meatballs with the mixture. Spray a large nonstick skillet with cooking spray and place over medium heat. Add the meatballs and cover. Cook until golden brown and juices run clear, about 5 minutes per side. If using a thermometer, cook until internal temperature reaches 165°F. Transfer to a serving plate and serve immediately.

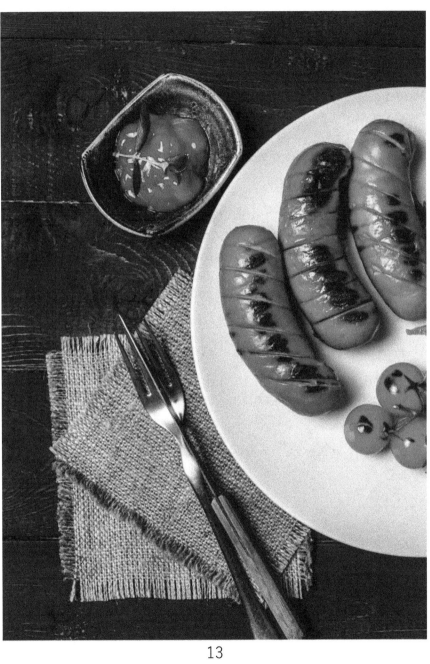

Papaya and Coconut Shake

Ready in about: 10 min
Serves: 2
Per serving:
Kcal 158, Sodium 40 mg, Protein 8 g, Carbs 26 g, Fat 3 g

INGREDIENTS:
- 1 ripe papaya, seeded, peeled, and cut into 1-inch chunks
- 1 cup plain low-fat yogurt
- 1 cup coconut water (not coconut milk)
- 2 tbsp. wheat germ
- ½ tsp. zero-calorie sweetener (optional)

DIRECTIONS:

Combine all ingredients, including sweetener (if using), in a blender. Pour into two tall glasses and serve.

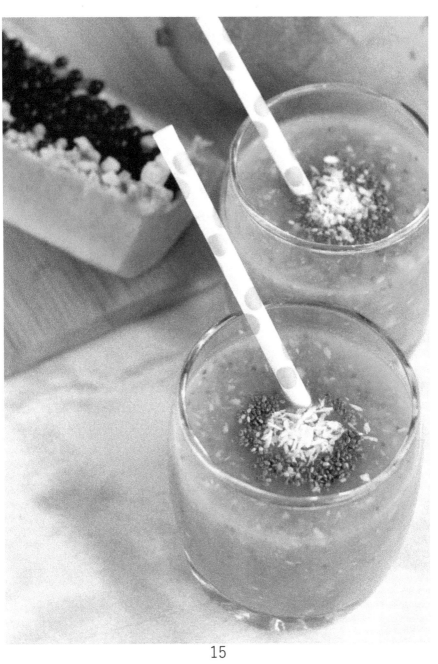

SOUPS AND CHOWDERS

Ingenious Eggplant Soup

Ready in about: 35 min
Serves: 4
Per serving:
Kcal 99, Sodium 163 mg, Protein 3.5 g, Carbs 7 g, Fat 7 g

INGREDIENTS:
- 1 large eggplant, washed and cubed
- 1 tomato, seeded and chopped
- 1 small onion, diced
- 2 tbsp. parsley, chopped
- 2 tbsp. extra virgin olive oil
- 2 tbsp. distilled white vinegar
- ½ cup parmesan cheese, crumbled
- Sunflower seeds as needed

DIRECTIONS:

Preheat your outdoor grill to medium-high heat. Punch the eggplant several times with a knife/fork. Cook the eggplants on the grill for about 15 minutes until they are charred. Set them aside and let them cool. Remove the skin from the eggplant and cut the pulp into cubes. Transfer the pulp to a bowl and add the parsley, onion, tomato, olive oil, parmesan cheese and vinegar. Mix well and let cool for 1 hour. Sprinkle with sunflower seeds and enjoy!

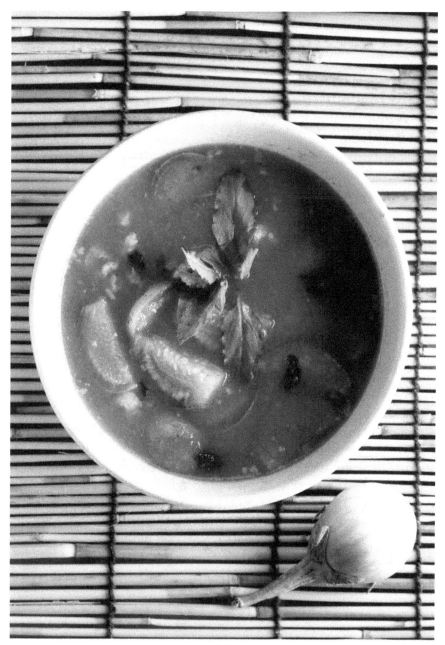

Low Sodium Vegetable Soup

Ready in about: 25 min
Serves: 3
Per serving:
Kcal 144, Sodium 102 mg, Protein 6.5 g, Carbs 28 g, Fat 0.5 g

INGREDIENTS:

- 3 cups low-sodium vegetable broth
- ½ cup spinach, chopped
- ⅓ cup broccoli, chopped
- 2 potatoes, chopped
- ¼ cup low-fat yogurt
- 2 oz. green beans, cooked
- 1 tsp. cayenne pepper
- 1 tomato, roughly chopped

DIRECTIONS:

Pour the broth inside the pot and bring it to a boil. Add the potatoes, cayenne pepper and green beans. Bring the ingredients to a boil and simmer for 5 minutes. Then add the spinach, yogurt, broccoli and tomato. Boil the soup for 10 minutes.

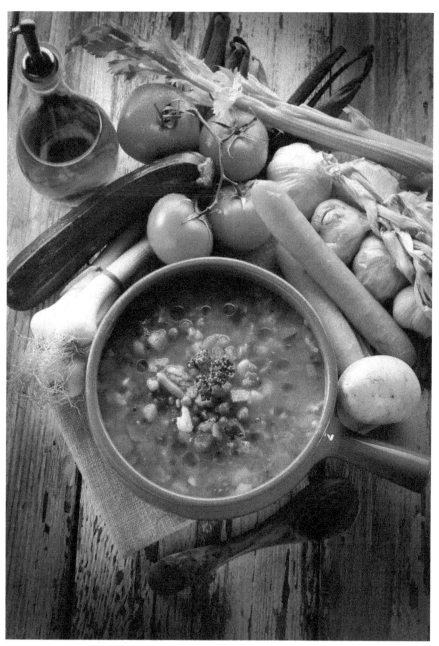

White Chicken Chilli

Ready in about: 50 min
Serves: 8
Per serving:
Kcal 212, Sodium 241 mg, Protein 19 g, Carbs 25 g, Fat 4 g

INGREDIENTS:

- 2 cans (15 oz. each) of low sodium white beans, drained
- 1 can (10 oz.) white chunk chicken
- 1 can (14.5 oz.) of low sodium diced tomatoes
- 1 medium onion, chopped
- 4 cups low-sodium chicken broth
- ½ medium green pepper, chopped
- 2 garlic cloves, minced
- 1 medium red pepper, chopped
- 2 tsp. chilli powder
- 1 tsp. dried oregano
- 1 tsp. ground cumin
- Cayenne pepper, to taste
- 3 tbsp. chopped fresh cilantro
- 8 tbsp. shredded reduced-fat Monterey Jack cheese

DIRECTIONS:

In a big pot, add the chicken, beans, tomatoes and chicken broth. Cover and cook over medium heat. Meanwhile, spray a nonstick skillet with cooking spray. Add onions, peppers and garlic and sauté until vegetables are tender, 3 to 5 minutes.

Include the onion and pepper mixture to the pot. Add the chilli powder, cumin, oregano and cayenne pepper to taste. Cook on low heat for approximate 10 minutes or until all the vegetables are tender. Pour into hot bowls. Sprinkle each serving with a tbsp. of cheese and garnish with cilantro. Serve hot.

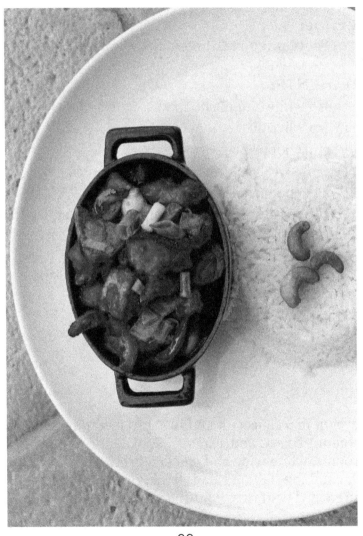

Wild Rice Mushroom Soup

Ready in about: 60 min
Serves: 4
Per serving:
Kcal 170, Sodium 120 mg, Protein 8 g, Carbs 23 g, Fat 5 g

INGREDIENTS:
- Half a white onion, chopped
- 1 tbsp. olive oil
- ¼ cup chopped celery
- 1½ cups of sliced fresh white mushrooms
- ¼ cup chopped carrots
- ½ cup of white wine, or ½ cup low-sodium, fat-free chicken broth
- 1 cup fat-free half-and-half
- 2½ cups of low-sodium, fat-free chicken broth
- 2 tbsp. flour
- Black pepper
- ¼ tsp. dried thyme
- 1 cup cooked wild rice

DIRECTIONS:

Put olive oil in a saucepan and bring to medium heat. Add the diced onion, celery and carrots. Cook until tender. Add the mushrooms, white wine and chicken broth. Cover and heat. In a bowl, combine half and half, flour, thyme and pepper. Then add the cooked wild rice. Pour the rice mixture into a saucepan with the vegetables. Cook over medium heat. Stir continuously until thick and bubbly and serve hot.

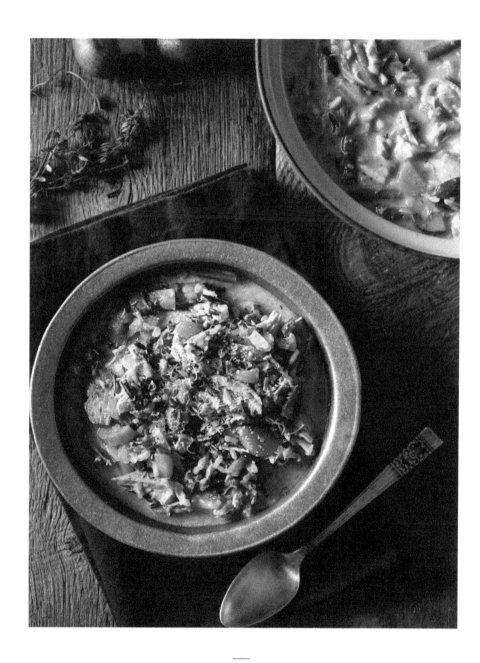

Zucchini Noodles Soup

Ready in about: 35 min
Serves: 4
Per serving:
Kcal 39, Sodium 158 mg, Protein 2 g, Carbs 5 g, Fat 1.5 g

INGREDIENTS:

- 2 zucchinis, trimmed
- 4 cups low-sodium chicken stock
- 2 oz. fresh parsley, chopped
- ½ tsp. chilli flakes
- 1 oz. carrot, shredded
- 1 tsp. canola oil

DIRECTIONS:

Grill the carrot with the canola oil in the pan for 5 minutes over medium-low heat. Mix well and add the chicken broth. Bring the mixture to a boil. Meanwhile, prepare the zucchini noodles using the spiralizer. Add them to the hot soup liquid. Add the parsley and chilli flakes. Bring the soup to a boil and take it away from the heat. Let it stand for 10 minutes. Serve.

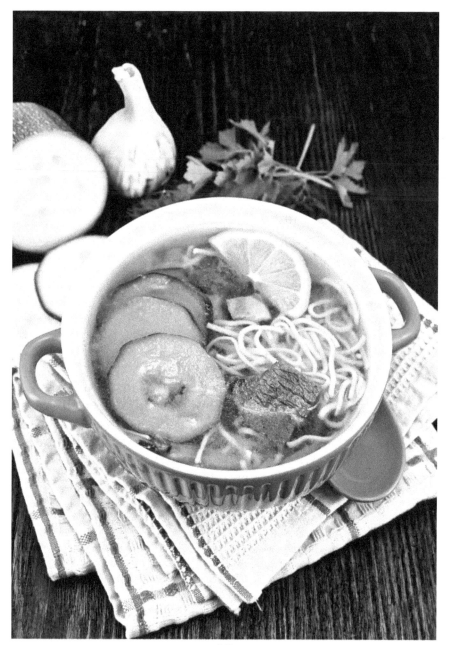

SALADS

Butternut Squash Apple Salad

Ready in about: 25 min
Serves: 6
Per serving:
Kcal: 215, Sodium 97 mg, Protein 5 g, Carbs 42 g, Fat 3 g

INGREDIENTS:

- 2 tsp. of olive oil
- A butternut squash, seeded and peeled, cut into ½ inch pieces
- 2 big apples, cored and cut ½-inch pieces
- 2 cups chopped carrots
- 1½ cups chopped celery
- 6 cups spinach, chopped
- 6 cups arugula, chopped

Dressing:

- ½ cup low-fat plain yogurt
- 2 tsp. balsamic vinegar
- 1½ tsp. honey

DIRECTIONS:

Heat oven to 400°F. Stirs squash in olive oil, roast in the oven for 20-30 minutes until golden and tender. Let it cool completely. Mix all the vegetables in a large bowl. Prepare the vinaigrette by mixing yogurt, vinegar and honey. Beat until smooth. Pour the vinaigrette over the salad. Toss and serve immediately with goat cheese and serve cold or at room temperature.

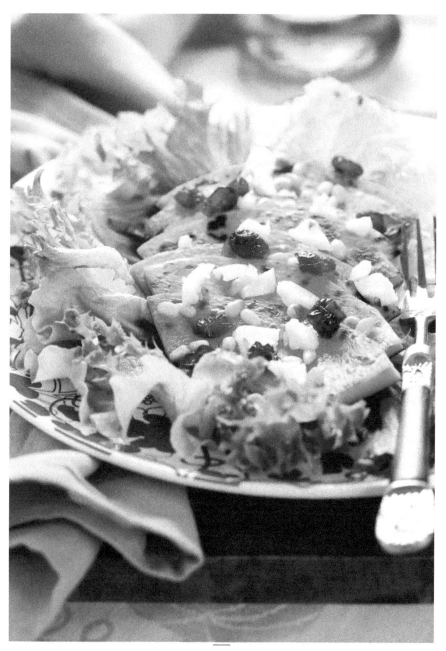

Corn Salad

Ready in about: 30 min
Serves: 4
Per serving:
Kcal 243, Sodium 153 mg, Protein 6 g, Carbs 43 g, Fat 7 g

INGREDIENTS:

- ¼ cup coarsely chopped cilantro
- 6 ears corn, shucked
- ¼ cup ¬nicely chopped red onion
- 2 roasted red bell peppers, diced (about 1 cup)
- 1-pint grape tomatoes, cut in half
- ¼ tsp. kosher salt
- Juice of 1 lime
- ¼ tsp. freshly ground black pepper
- 1½ tbsp. extra-virgin olive oil

DIRECTIONS:

In an enormous pot of boiling water, cook the ears of corn until the kernels have turned bright yellow, 3 to 4 minutes. Drain and let cool. When cool enough to handle, remove the corn kernels from the cob using a knife. Put the corn in a large bowl, and add the cilantro, red onion, tomatoes, bell peppers, salt, black pepper, lime juice, and olive oil. Mix the salad, taste, and adjust the seasonings as needed. Serve.

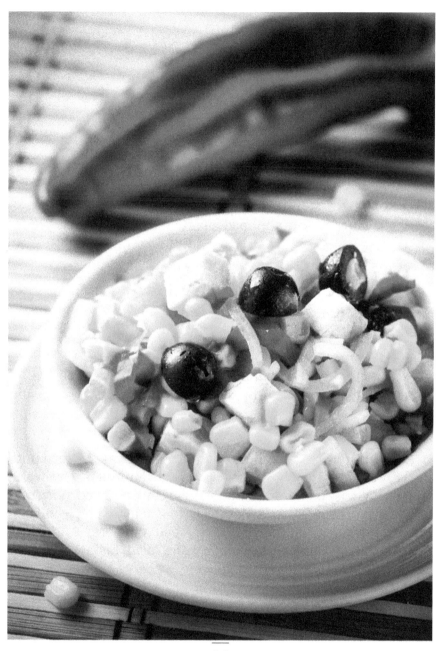

Mango Tango Salad

Ready in about: 20 min
Serves: 6
Per serving:
Kcal 68, Sodium 10 mg, Protein 1 g, Carbs 16 g, Fat 0.5 g

INGREDIENTS:

- 3 ripe mangoes, pitted and cubed
- Juice of 1 lime
- 1 tsp. minced red onion
- 2 tbsp. chopped of fresh cilantro leaves
- ½ jalapeno pepper, seeded and minced

DIRECTIONS:

Combine all ingredients in a mixing bowl. Let stand 10 minutes. Toss just before serving.

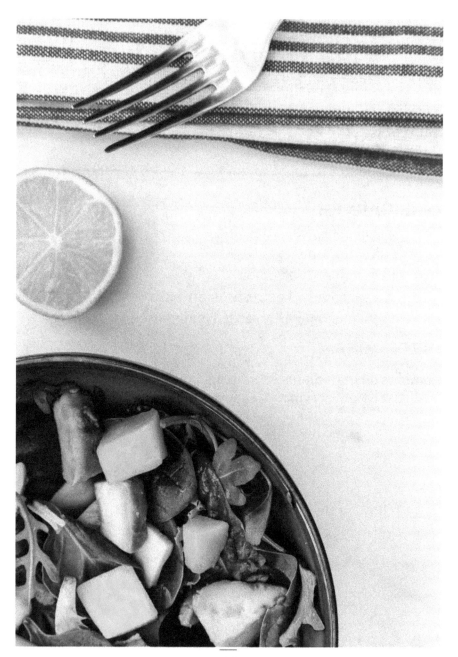

Watermelon Shrimp Salad

Ready in about: 1 h 15 min
Serves: 4
Per serving:
Kcal 234, Sodium 696 mg, Protein 17 g, Carbs 23 g, Fat 9 g

INGREDIENTS:

- Olive oil in a pump sprayer

- 1-pound large shrimp (21 to 25), peeled and deveined
- 6 cups seedless watermelon cubes, cut into 1-inch squares, chilled
- ½ medium red onion, cut into thin half-moons
- 24 large basil leaves, cut into thin shreds (¼ cup packed)
- 1 recipe Lime Vinaigrette

DIRECTIONS:

Spray a large nonstick skillet with oil and heat over medium-high heat. Add the shrimp and cook, occasionally stirring, until completely opaque, about 3 minutes. Move it to a plate and leave it to cool. Cover and refrigerate until chilled, at least 1 hour. In a large serving bowl, combine the watermelon, onion and basil. Add the shrimp and the vinaigrette and mix gently. Serve cold.

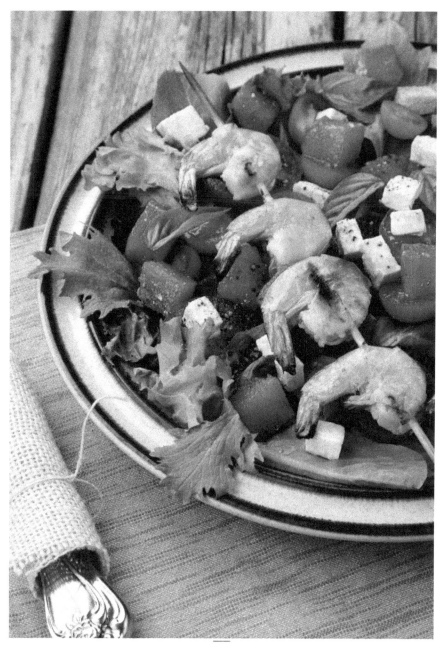

PLANT-BASED MAINS

Corn Patties

Ready in about: 25 min
Serves: 4
Per serving:
Kcal 168, Sodium 23 mg, Protein 6.5 g, Carbs 25 g, Fat 6 g

INGREDIENTS:
- ½ cup chickpeas, cooked
- 1 cup corn kernels, cooked
- 1 tbsp. fresh parsley, chopped
- 1 tsp. chili powder
- ½ tsp. ground coriander
- 1 tbsp. tomato paste
- 1 tbsp. almond meal
- 1 tbsp. olive oil

DIRECTIONS:

Crush the cooked chickpeas and combine them with the corn kernels, parsley, chili powder, ground cilantro, tomato paste, and almond meal. Stir the mixture until it is smooth. Prepare the patties. Then heat the olive oil in the pan. Place prepared patties in boiling oil and cook for 3 minutes per side or until golden brown. Pat the cooked patties dry with a paper towel if necessary. Serve.

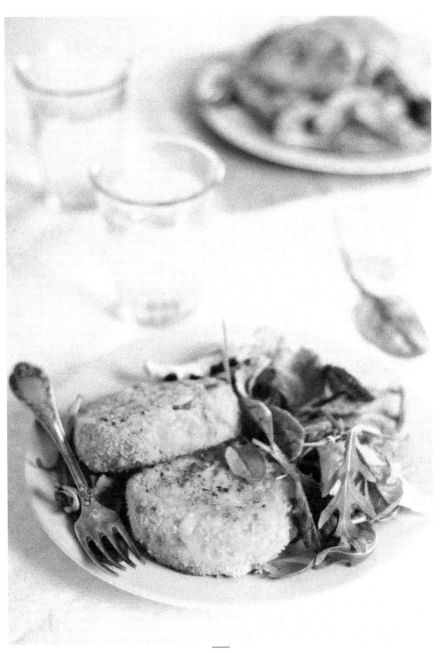

Tofu Stir Fry

Ready in about: 25 min
Serves: 3
Per serving:
Kcal 118, Sodium 406 mg, Protein 8.5 g, Carbs 3 g, Fat 8.5 g

INGREDIENTS:

- 9 oz. firm tofu, cubed
- 3 tbsp. low-sodium soy sauce
- 1 tsp. sesame seeds
- 1 tbsp. sesame oil
- 1 cup spinach, chopped
- ¼ cup of water

DIRECTIONS:

In the bowl, combine the soy sauce and sesame oil. Dip the tofu cubes in the soy sauce mixture and marinate for 10 minutes. Heat a skillet and put the tofu cubes in it. Cook them for 1.5 minutes on each side. Then add the water, the rest of the soy sauce mixture, and the chopped spinach. Close the lid and cook the flour for another 5 minutes. Serve.

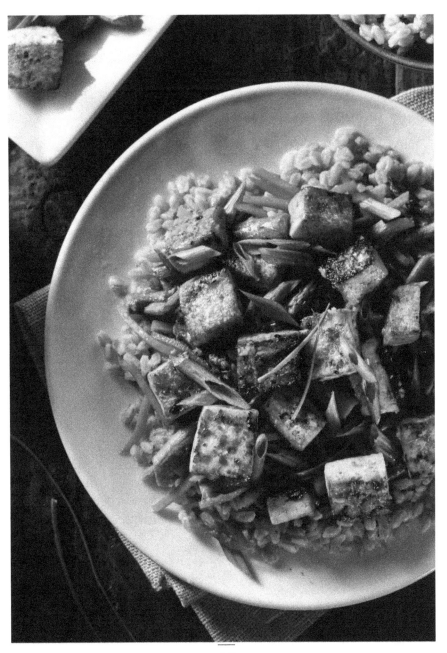

Tofu Tikka Masala

Ready in about: 35 min
Serves: 2
Per serving:
Kcal 155, Sodium 51 mg, Protein 12 g, Carbs 20.5 g, Fat 8.5 g

INGREDIENTS:

- 8 oz. tofu, chopped
- ½ cup of soy milk
- 1 tsp. garam masala
- 1 tsp. olive oil
- 1 tsp. ground paprika
- ½ cup tomatoes, chopped
- ½ onion, diced

DIRECTIONS:

Heat the olive oil in the pan. Add the chopped onion to the already heated oil and cook until golden brown. Then add the tomatoes, ground paprika, and garam masala. Bring the mixture to a boil. Add soy milk and mix well. Simmer for 5 minutes. Then add the chopped tofu and cook the food for 3 minutes. Let the cooked food rest for 10 minutes and serve.

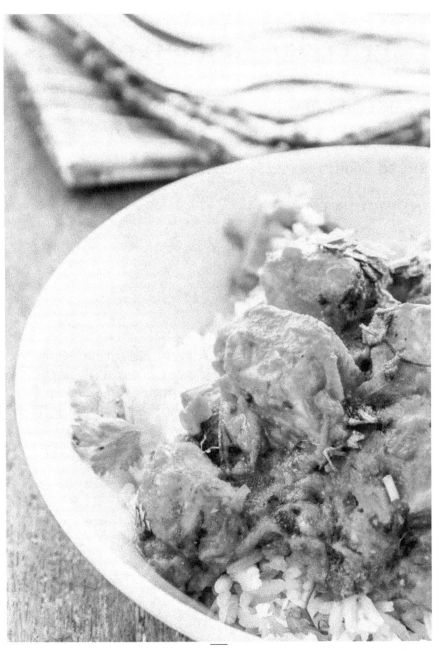

Turmeric Cauliflower Florets

Ready in about: 35 min
Serves: 4
Per serving:
Kcal 50, Sodium 16 mg, Protein 1 g, Carbs 4.5 g, Fat 4 g

INGREDIENTS:
- 2 cups cauliflower florets
- 1 tbsp. ground turmeric
- 1 tsp. smoked paprika
- 1 tbsp. olive oil

DIRECTIONS:

Sprinkle the cauliflower florets with ground turmeric, smoked paprika, and olive oil. Then line the pot with baking paper and place the cauliflower florets in the pan in a single layer. Cook the food for 25 minutes at 375°F or until the cauliflower florets are tender. Serve immediately.

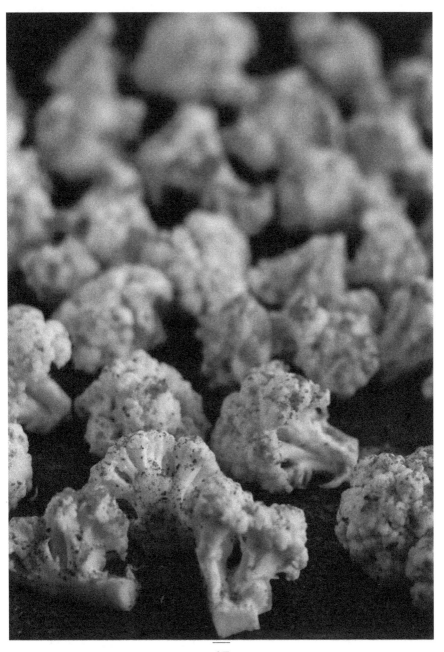

Vegetarian Kebabs

Ready in about: 16 min
Serves: 4
Per serving:
Kcal 88, Sodium 14 mg, Protein 2.5 g, Carbs 4 g, Fat 4 g

INGREDIENTS:

- 2 tbsp. balsamic vinegar
- 1 tbsp. olive oil
- 1 tsp. dried parsley
- 2 tbsp. water
- 2 sweet peppers
- 2 red onions, peeled
- 2 zucchinis, trimmed

DIRECTIONS:

Cut the sweet peppers and onions into medium squares. Then cut the zucchini. Put all the vegetables on the skewers. Then, in a shallow bowl, combine the olive oil, dried parsley, water, and balsamic vinegar. Sprinkle the vegetable skewers with the olive oil mixture and transfer to a preheated 390°F grill. Cook the skewers on both side for 3 minutes, or until the vegetables are golden brown. Serve immediately.

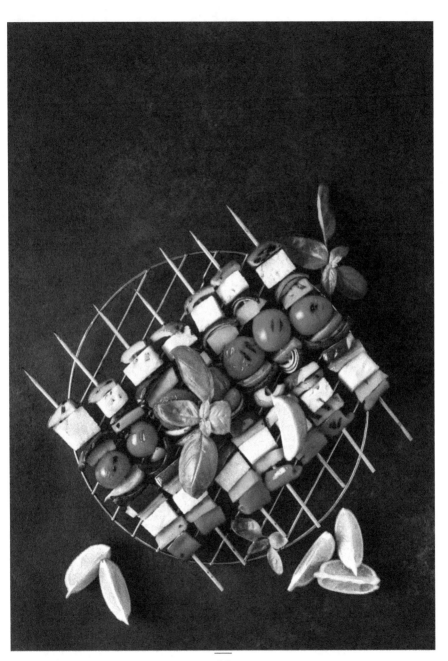

Vegetarian Lasagna

Ready in about: 40 min
Serves: 6
Per serving:
Kcal 77, Sodium 113 mg, Protein 4.5 g, Carbs 9.5 g, Fat 3 g

INGREDIENTS:
- 1 cup carrot, diced
- ½ cup bell pepper, diced
- 1 cup spinach, chopped
- 1 tbsp. olive oil
- 1 tsp. chili powder
- 1 cup tomatoes, chopped
- 4 oz. low-fat cottage cheese
- 1 eggplant, sliced
- 1 cup low-sodium chicken broth

DIRECTIONS:

Place the carrot, pepper, and spinach in the pot. Add olive oil and chili powder and mix the vegetables well. Cook them for 5 minutes. Then place the sliced eggplant layer in the casserole dish and garnish with the vegetable mixture. Add the tomatoes and cottage cheese. Bake the lasagna for 30 minutes at 375°F. Serve hot.

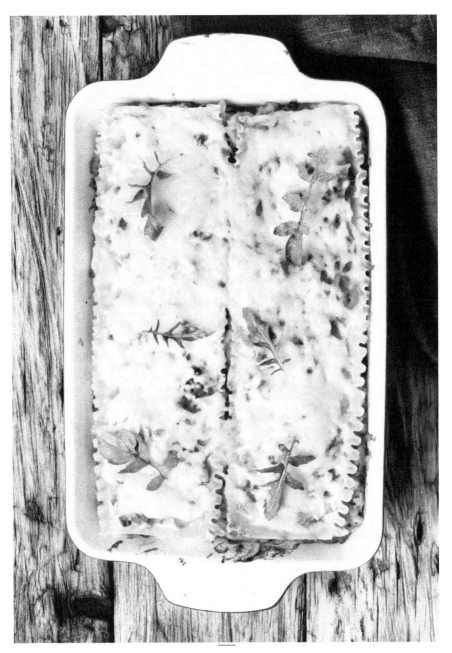

POULTRY

Chicken Sliders

Ready in about: 30 min
Serves: 4
Per serving:
Kcal 224, Sodium 173 mg, Protein 22 g, Carbs 25 g, Fat 4 g

INGREDIENTS:
- 10 oz. ground chicken breast
- 1 tbsp. black pepper
- 1 tbsp. minced garlic
- 1 tbsp. balsamic vinegar
- ½ cup minced onion
- 1 fresh chili pepper, minced
- 1 tbsp. fennel seed, crushed
- 4 whole-wheat mini buns
- 4 lettuce leaves
- 4 tomato slices

DIRECTIONS:

Mix the first 7 items and refrigerate for 1 hour. Form into 4 patties. Roast or broil in the oven until it reaches a minimum internal temperature of 165°F. Serve on small whole-wheat buns with lettuce and tomatoes.

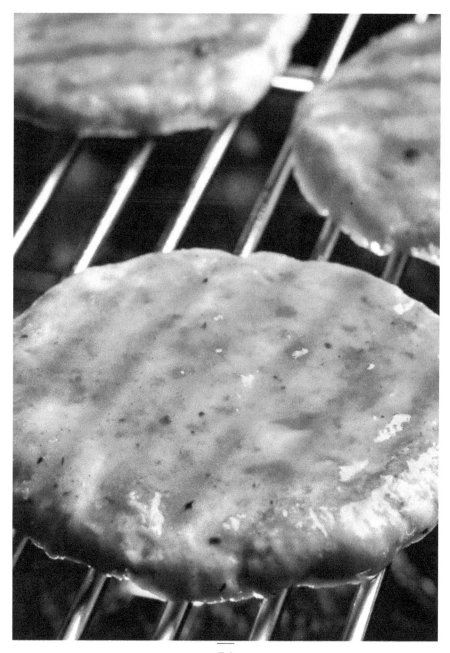

Chicken with Paprika Scallions

Ready in about: 40 min
Serves: 4
Per serving:
Kcal 295, Sodium 200 mg, Protein 15 g, Carbs 22 g, Fat 12.5 g

INGREDIENTS:

- 4 scallions, chopped
- 1 pound chicken breast, skinless, boneless and sliced
- 1 tbsp. olive oil
- 1 cup low-sodium chicken stock
- 1 tbsp. sweet paprika
- 1 tbsp. ginger, grated
- 1 tsp. cumin, ground
- 1 tsp. oregano, dried
- 1 tsp. allspice, ground
- A pinch of black pepper
- ½ cup cilantro, chopped

DIRECTIONS:

Warmth a pan with the oil over medium heat, add the scallions and the meat and brown for 5 minutes. Add the rest of the ingredients, toss, introduce in the oven and bake at 390°F for 25 minutes. Divide the chicken and scallions, mix between plates and serve.

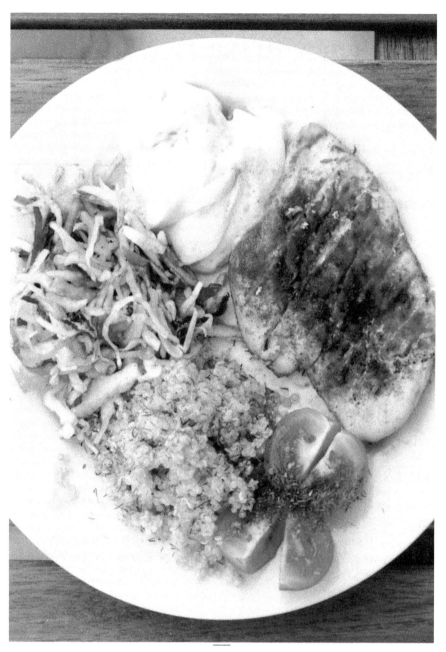

Chicken with Red Onion Mix

Ready in about: 35 min
Serves: 4
Per serving:
Kcal 364, Sodium 160 mg, Protein 41.5 g, Carbs 9 g, Fat 17.5 g

INGREDIENTS:

- 3 red onions, sliced
- 2 chicken breasts, skinless, boneless and roughly cubed
- 2 tbsp. olive oil
- 1 tbsp. chives, chopped
- A pinch of black pepper
- 1 cup low-sodium veggie stock
- 1 tbsp. cilantro, chopped

DIRECTIONS:

Warmth a pan with the oil over medium heat, add the onions and a pinch of black pepper and sauté for 10 minutes, stirring often. Include the chicken and cook for 3 minutes more. Add the rest of the ingredients, bring to a simmer and cook over medium heat for 12 minutes more. Divide the chicken and onions mix between plates and serve.

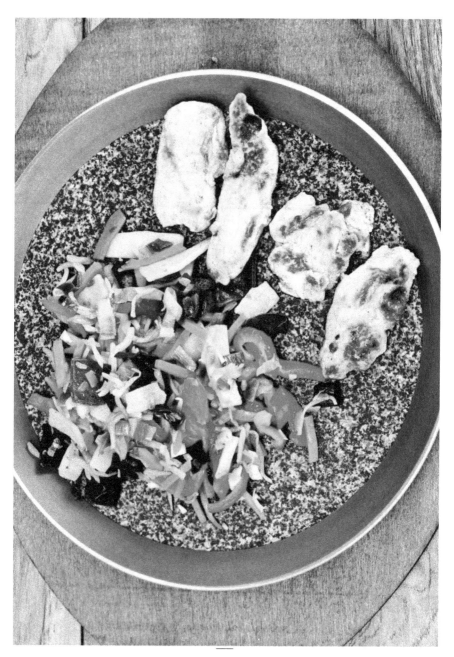

Chipotle Chicken

Ready in about: 1 h 10 min
Serves: 6
Per serving:
Kcal 280, Sodium 369.5 mg, Protein 12 g, Carbs 15 g, Fat 12 g

INGREDIENTS:
- 1 yellow onion, chopped
- 2 pounds chicken thighs, boneless and skinless
- 2 tbsp. olive oil
- 1 tbsp. coriander seeds, ground
- 3 garlic cloves, minced
- 1 tsp. cumin, ground
- 1 tbsp. coriander, chopped
- 4 tbsp. chipotle chili paste
- 1 cup low-sodium chicken stock
- A pinch of black pepper

DIRECTIONS:

Warmth a pan with the oil over medium heat, add the onion and the garlic and sauté for 5 minutes. Add the meat and brown for 5 minutes more. Add the rest of the ingredients, toss, introduce everything in the oven and bake at 390°F for 50 minutes. Divide the whole mix between plates and serve.

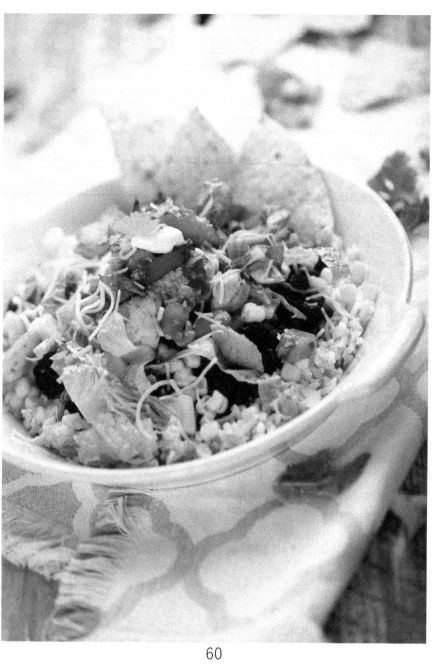

Cinnamon Roasted Chicken

Ready in about: 2 h
Serves: 4
Per serving:
Kcal 329, Sodium 387 mg, Protein 19 g, Carbs 19 g, Fat 14 g

INGREDIENTS:
- 2 tbsp. unsalted butter, at room temperature
- 3 Red Delicious apples, sliced
- 2 tsp. of grated orange zest (about 1 orange)
- 1 (3¼ to 3½-pound) whole chicken
- ½ tsp. kosher salt
- 1 tsp. ground cinnamon
- ¼ tsp. freshly ground black pepper

DIRECTIONS:

Preheat the oven to 425°F. Spread the apples in the baking dish. Combine the butter, orange zest, cinnamon, salt, and pepper in a small bowl. Rinse the chicken and blot dry. Using a knife, cut the backbone out. Place the chicken split-side down on top of the apples. Divide the butter mixture into two and rub half underneath the skin. Rub the remaining half on the skin. Cook the chicken until the temperature reaches 180°F, or the juices run clear when pricked, about 40 minutes. Tent the chicken with aluminum foil to keep warm and let rest for about 5 minutes. Cut the chicken into pieces and serve with the roasted apples and juices.

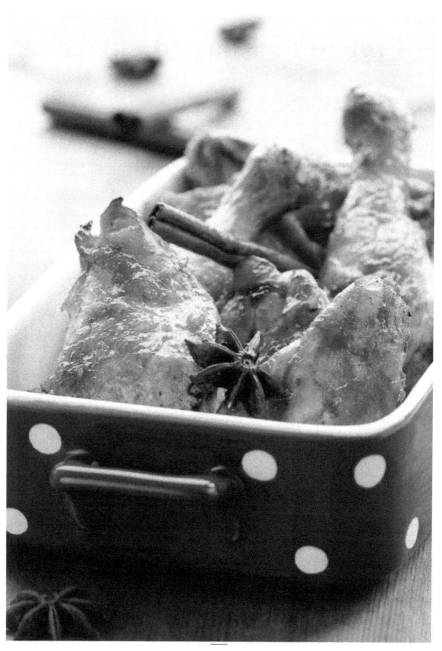

FISH AND SEAFOOD

Fish Spread

Ready in about: 10 min
Serves: 8
Per serving:
Kcal 231, Sodium 90 mg, Protein 31 g, Carbs 1 g, Fat 10.5 g

INGREDIENTS:

- 2-pounds trout, boiled
- 2 tbsp. low-fat cream cheese
- 1 tbsp. fresh dill, chopped
- 1 tsp. minced garlic
- ¼ cup low-fat yogurt

DIRECTIONS:

Put all the ingredients together in the food processor and mix until smooth. Transfer the fish spread to the bowl and flatten well. Refrigerate the spread for 5 to 10 minutes before serving.

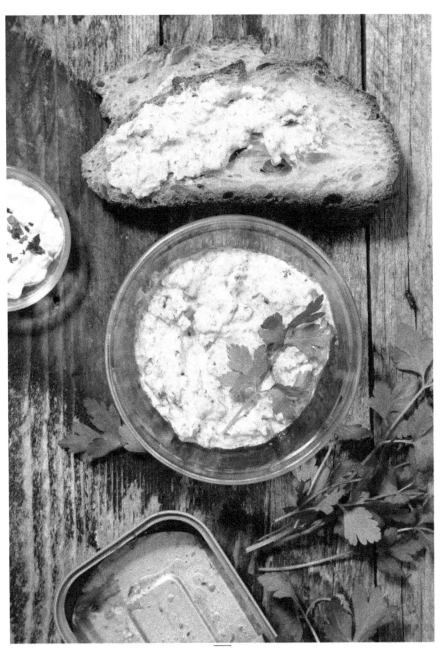

Herbed Sole

Ready in about: 20 min
Serves: 3
Per serving:
Kcal 185, Sodium 191 mg, Protein 23.5 g, Carbs 1.5 g, Fat 9 g

INGREDIENTS:

- 10 oz. sole fillet
- 2 tbsp. margarine
- 1 tbsp. dill weed
- 1 tsp. garlic powder
- ½ tsp. cumin seeds

DIRECTIONS:

Put the margarine in the saucepan. Add the cumin seeds and dill weed. Melt the mixture and simmer for 30 seconds. Then cut the sole fillet into 2 portions and sprinkle with garlic powder. Place the fish fillets in the melted margarine mixture. Cook the fish for three minutes on each side.

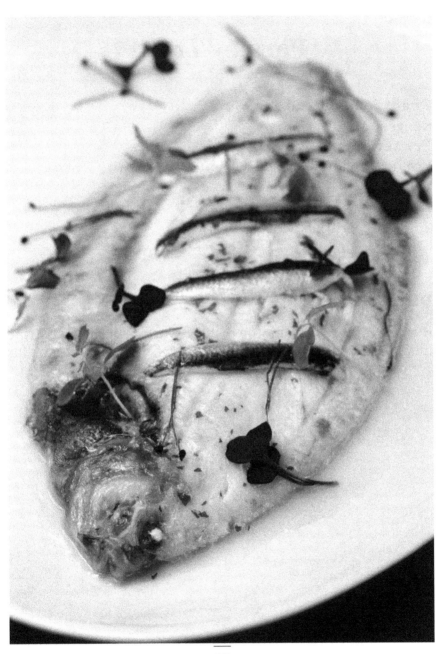

Parsley Trout

Ready in about: 20 min
Serves: 4
Per serving:
Kcal 152, Sodium 86 mg, Protein 16.5 g, Carbs 0 g, Fat 9 g

INGREDIENTS:
- 1 tbsp. dried parsley
- 6 trout fillets
- 2 tbsp. margarine

DIRECTIONS:

Rub the trout fillets with the parsley. Then pour the margarine into the saucepan and melt. Include the fish fillets and cook for 4 minutes per side. Serve warm.

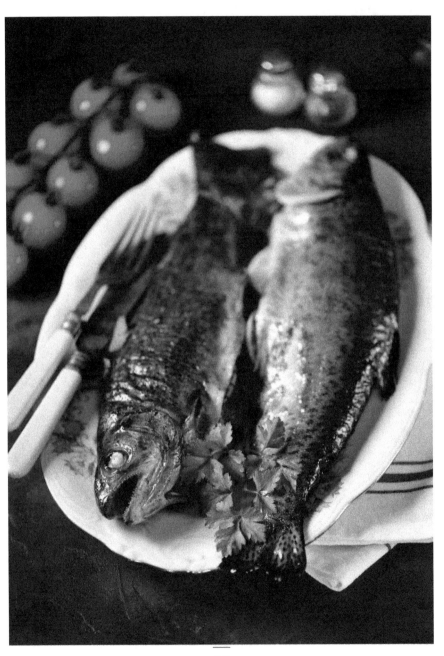

Spiced Scallops

Ready in about: 15 min
Serves: 4
Per serving:
Kcal 130, Sodium 195 mg, Protein 19 g, Carbs 2.5 g, Fat 4.5 g

INGREDIENTS:
- 1-pound scallops
- 1 tsp. Cajun seasonings
- 1 tbsp. olive oil

DIRECTIONS:

Rub the scallops with the Cajun seasonings. Heat the olive oil in the pan. Add the scallops and cook for 2 minutes per side.

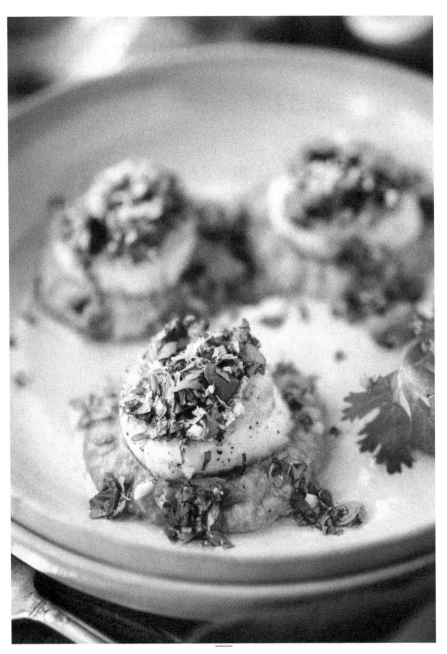

Tuna and Pineapple Kebob

Ready in about: 18 min
Serves: 4
Per serving:
Kcal 347, Sodium 1 mg, Protein 18 g, Carbs 7.5 g, Fat 27.5 g

INGREDIENTS:
- 12 oz. tuna fillet
- 8 oz. pineapple, peeled
- 1 tsp. olive oil
- ¼ tsp. ground fennel

DIRECTIONS:

Chop the tuna and pineapple into medium cubes and sprinkle with olive oil and ground fennel. Then put them on the skewers and place them on the grill preheated to 400°F. Cook the kebobs for 4 minutes per side. Serve.

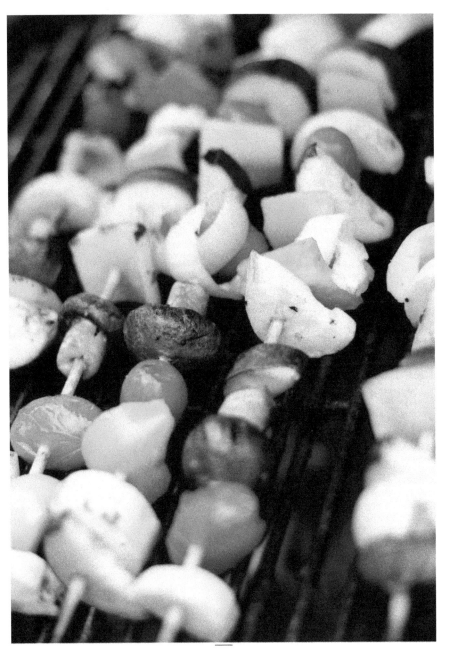

Turmeric Pate

Ready in about: 18 min
Serves: 6
Per serving:
Kcal 149, Sodium 46 mg, Protein 20.5 g, Carbs 1 g, Fat 6.5 g

INGREDIENTS:

- 1-pound tuna, canned
- 3 tsp. lemon juice
- ¼ cup low-fat yogurt
- 1 tsp. ground cinnamon
- ½ tsp. ground turmeric

DIRECTIONS:

Blend he ingredients together in the food processor. Mix the pâté until smooth and transfer to the bowl.

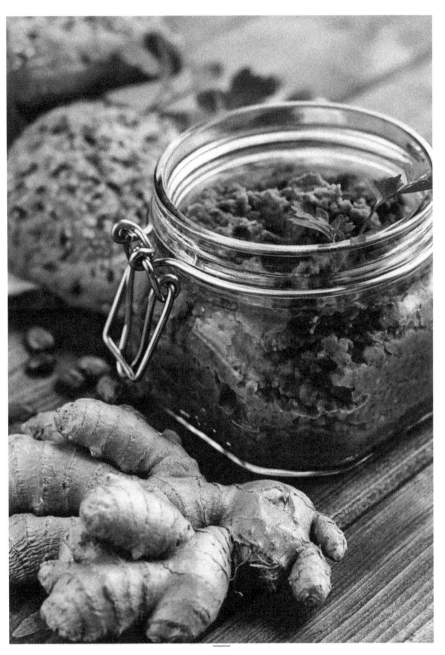

SIDE DISHES

Creamed Swiss Chard

Ready in about: 25 min
Serves: 8
Per serving:
Kcal 80, Sodium 265 mg, Protein 3 g, Carbs 8 g, Fat 4 g

INGREDIENTS:
- 2 tbsp. olive oil
- 1½ tbsp. unbleached all-purpose flour
- 3 garlic cloves, finely chopped
- 1¼ cups low-fat plain soy milk
- 2 pounds Swiss chard, washed, stemmed and cut crosswise into strips ½ inch wide
- ½ tsp. freshly ground black pepper
- 1 tbsp. grated Parmesan cheese

DIRECTIONS:

In a big size skillet, heat up the olive oil over medium heat. Incorporate the flour to obtain a homogeneous dough. Continue to beat and add the garlic; cook for another 30 seconds. Add the soy milk and cook until the mixture thickens a little. Add the chard and toss to coat them well. Cover the lid and cook until tender, about 2 minutes. Season with pepper. Sprinkle with Parmesan and serve hot.

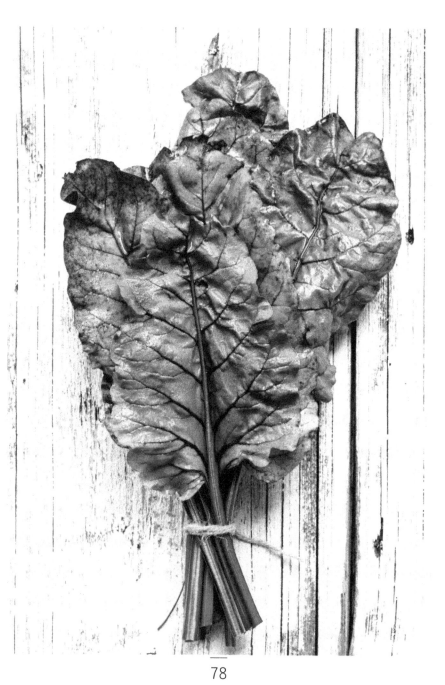

Roasted Winter Squash

Ready in about: 1 h 15 min
Serves: 8
Per serving:
Kcal 184, Sodium 6 mg, Protein 5.5 g, Carbs 32 g, Fat 4 g

INGREDIENTS:

- 2 tsp. canola oil, divided
- 4 cups of peeled and diced (½-inch pieces) winter squash
- 1 cup diced onion
- 4 cups cooked wild rice
- 1 cup fresh cranberries
- ¼ cup walnuts, chopped
- Black pepper to taste
- ½ tbsp. chopped Italian parsley
- 1 small orange, peeled and segmented
- ¼ tsp. thyme

DIRECTIONS:

Heat up the oven to 400°F. Place the squash in the pan and season with 1 tsp. of oil. Bake for 40 minutes or until golden brown. In a hot skillet, brown the onions with the remaining oil. Add the cranberries and sauté for 1 minute. Add remaining ingredients and sauté for 4 to 5 minutes or until heated through. Serve.

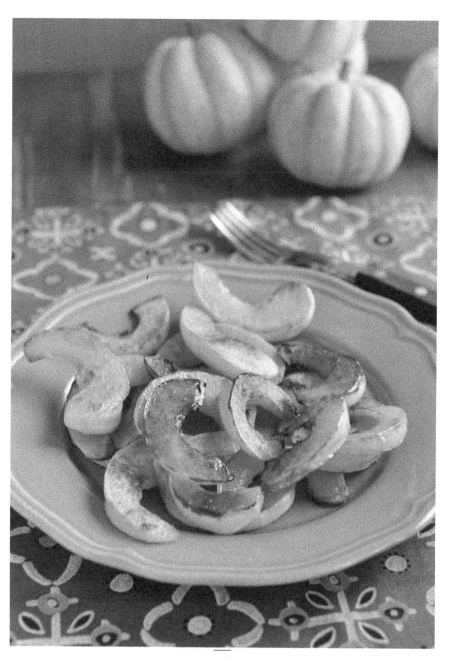

Seared Endive

Ready in about: 30 min
Serves: 4
Per serving:
Kcal 24, Sodium 150 mg, Protein 1 g, Carbs 5 g, Fat 0 g

INGREDIENTS:

- 1 tbsp. water
- 8 heads of Belgian endive, washed and halved
- Juice from 1 lemon
- ¼ tsp. salt
- Ground black pepper, if desired
- 2 tbsp. chopped fresh parsley

DIRECTIONS:

In a large skillet, heat the water over medium heat. Add the endives, cut sides down. Cover the lid and cook for several minutes until the outer leaves become translucent. Remove from the heat and uncover. Squeeze the lemon juice over the endive and season with pepper. Transfer to a serving platter and garnish with parsley. Serve immediately.

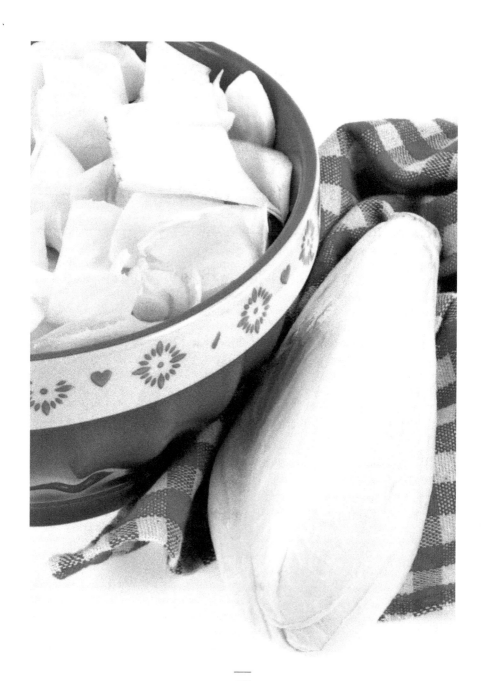

Sweet Carrots

Ready in about: 25 min
Serves: 4
Per serving:
Kcal 148, Sodium 35 mg, Protein 3 g, Carbs 34 g, Fat 0.5 g

INGREDIENTS:
- ½ cup water
- ¼ tsp. salt
- 2 cups shredded carrots
- 1 tsp. trans-free margarine
- The sugar substitute, to taste
- 1 tsp. lemon juice
- 4 tbsp. fresh parsley, chopped

DIRECTIONS:

In a portable saucepan, bring the water to a boil. Add salt and chopped carrots. Cover the lid and cook until the water has evaporated, about 5 minutes. Remove the carrots from the heat. Add the margarine, sugar substitute, lemon juice and parsley. Serve immediately.

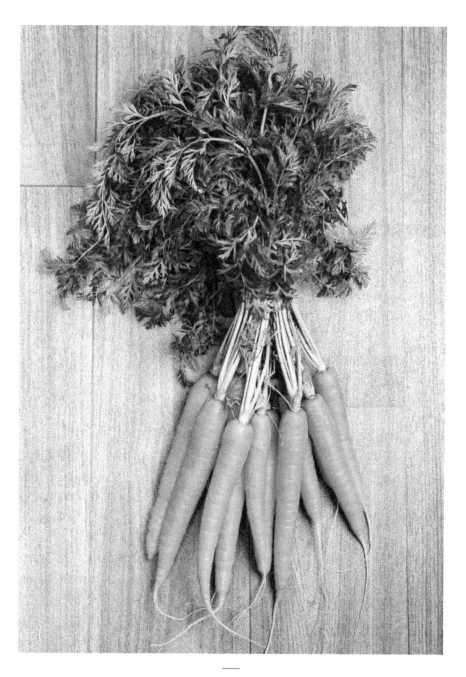

SNACKS

Crunchy Garbanzo Bean

Ready in about: 50 min
Serves: 8
Per serving:
Kcal 56, Sodium 56 mg, Protein 3 g, Carbs 10 g, Fat 1 g

INGREDIENTS:

- 1 tsp. fresh dill
- 1 tsp. fresh parsley
- 2 cans unsalted garbanzo beans
- 1 tsp. crushed garlic

DIRECTIONS:

Preheat the oven to 350°F. Make a baking tray with cooking spray in a mixing bowl, put the drained beans and toss with fresh dill, crushed garlic, onion powder, salt, parsley, and pepper. Give the mixture a good toss, then pour it into the baking tray. Place the baking tray in the oven and cook for 35 to 40 minutes. The beans should be crisp and bloated. Spurt them into a bowl and allow them to cool. Serve and eat as or when needed.

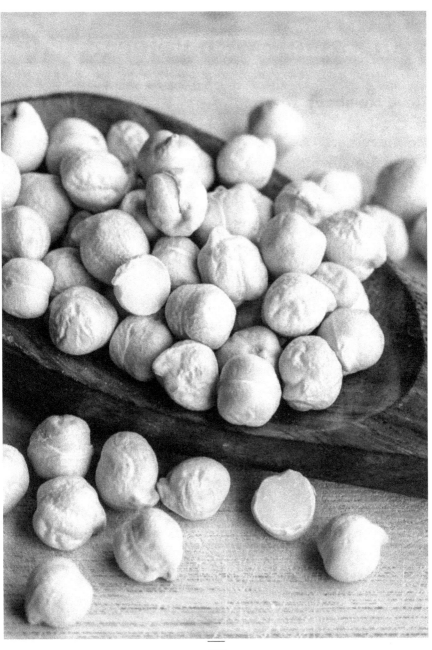

Guacamole with Pomegranate

Ready in about: 20 min
Serves: 4
Per serving:
Kcal 173, Sodium 154 mg, Protein 2 g, Carbs 11 g, Fat 7 g

INGREDIENTS:
- 2 tbsp. chopped cilantro
- 2 ripe avocados, diced
- 1 scallion, chopped
- Multigrain tortilla chips, to serve
- ¼ tsp. kosher salt
- Juice of ½ lime
- ¼ cup pomegranate seeds

DIRECTIONS:

In a portable bowl, mash the avocado using a fork. Add the cilantro, scallion, lime juice, salt, and half the pomegranate seeds and mix. Top with the remaining pomegranate seeds and serve with tortilla chips.

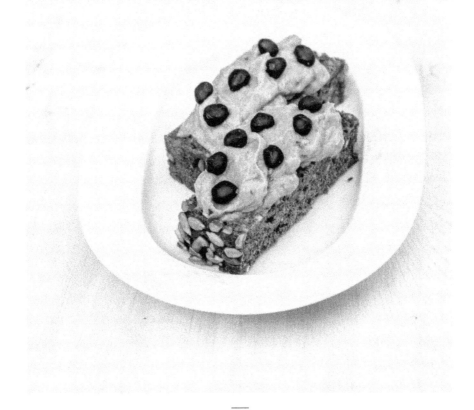

Honey Orange Sauce

Ready in about: 25 min
Serves: 4
Per serving:
Kcal 96, Sodium 4 mg, Protein 1 g, Carbs 24 g, Fat 1 g

INGREDIENTS:
- 2 tbsp. lemon juice
- ⅓ cup unsweetened orange juice
- 1½ tbsp. honey
- 1 dash nutmeg
- ¼ tsp. ground ginger

DIRECTIONS:

Prepare the fruit. Combine all ingredients for sauce and mix. Pour honey–orange sauce over fruit.

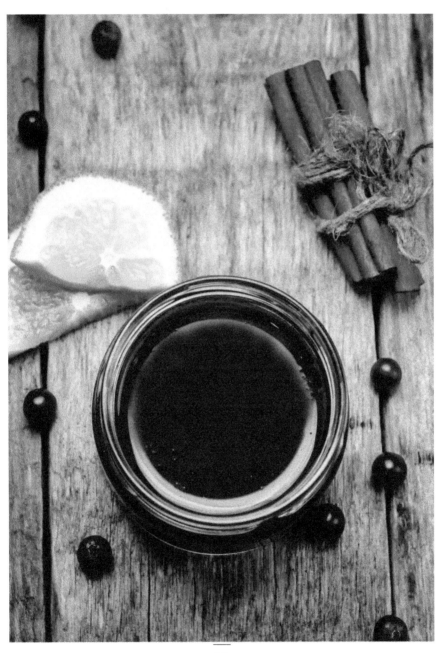

Potato Casserole

Ready in about: 30 min
Serves: 10
Per serving:
Kcal 237, Sodium 22.5 mg, Protein 6 g, Carbs 47 g, Fat 3 g

INGREDIENTS:

- ¼ tsp. black pepper
- 1 tsp. dried dill weed
- ¼ cup green onions, chopped
- 16 small new potatoes, around 5 cups
- 2 tbsp. olive oil

DIRECTIONS:

Using water and vegetable brush clean all potatoes. For about 20 minutes, boil potatoes then drain and cool them for 20 minutes. Mix spices, onions, and olive oil. Then cut potatoes into quarters and combine with the mixture. Refrigerate and enjoy!

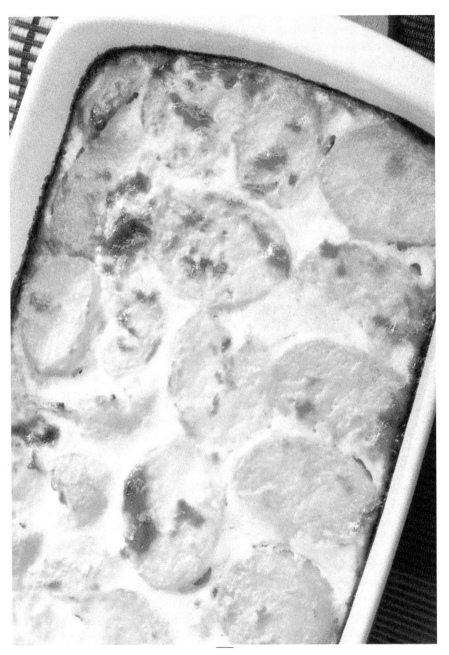

Trail Mix

Ready in about: 15 min
Serves: 4
Per serving:
Kcal 156, Sodium 76 mg, Protein 4 g, Carbs 21 g, Fat 7 g

INGREDIENTS:
- ¼ cup unsalted dry-roasted peanuts
- ¼ cup whole shelled (unpeeled) almonds
- ¼ cup dried cranberries
- 2 oz. dried apricots, or other dried fruit
- ¼ cup chopped pitted dates

DIRECTIONS:

Mix all the ingredients together and enjoy.

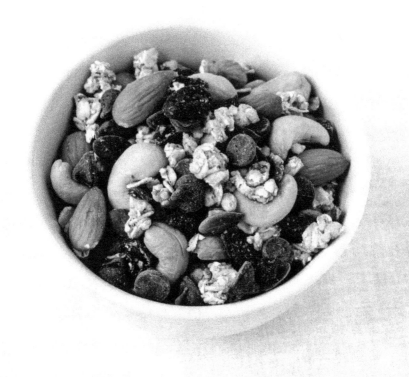

DESSERTS

Peach Floats

Ready in about: 60 min
Serves: 4
Per serving:
Kcal 233, Sodium 189 mg, Protein 7 g, Carbs 49 g, Fat 1 g

INGREDIENTS:

- 4 cups vanilla ice milk
- 1 can (15 oz.) of peaches, drained, except for ½ cup juice
- 32 oz. club soda or seltzer water
- Ground nutmeg, to taste
- ½ cup reduced-fat whipped topping

DIRECTIONS:

In a portable bowl, mash the peaches with a fork. Divide the peach puree among 4 glasses (12 oz. each). Add 2 tbsp. of peach juice and 1 cup of ice milk to each glass. Pour 1 cup of soda or seltzer into the glasses. Garnish each drink with 2 tbsp. of whipped topping and a pinch of nutmeg. Serve immediately.

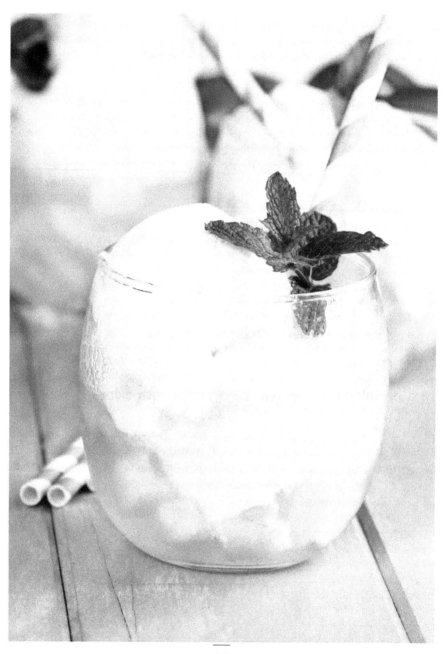

Pumpkin Cream Cheese Dip

Ready in about: 10 min
Serves: 12
Per serving:
Kcal 99, Sodium 69 mg, Protein 2 g, Carbs 10 g, Fat 3 g

INGREDIENTS:

- ¾ cup of unsweetened and unsalted canned pumpkin
- 8 oz. low-fat cream cheese (room temperature)
- 3 tbsp. sugar
- ¼ tsp. nutmeg
- ½ tsp. cinnamon
- ¼ tsp. ground cloves
- 6 apples, sliced
- ½ tsp. vanilla

DIRECTIONS:

Combine all the cream ingredients in a bowl by hand or with an electric mixer (medium speed). Serve with apple slices for dipping.

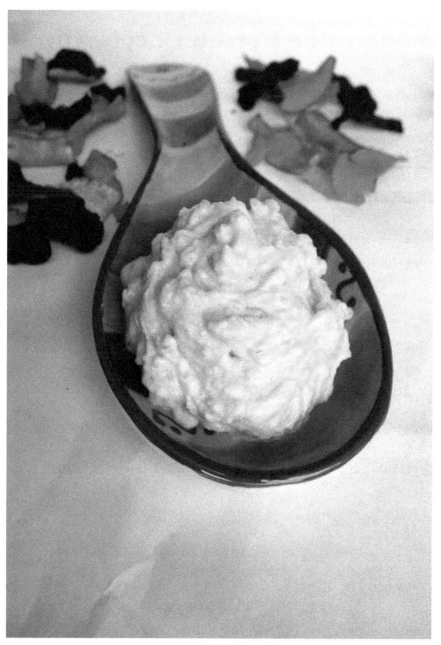

Rainbow Ice Pops

Ready in about: 2 h
Serves: 6
Per serving:
Kcal 60, Sodium 6 mg, Protein 0.5 g, Carbs 14 g, Fat 0.5 g

INGREDIENTS:
- ½ cup blueberries
- 1½ cups diced strawberries, watermelon and cantaloupe
- 2 cups 100% apple juice
- 6 craft sticks
- 6 paper cups (6-8 oz. each)

DIRECTIONS:

Mix the fruits together and distribute them evenly among the paper cups. For each paper cup, pour in ⅓ cup of juice. Place the cups in the freezer on a flat surface. Freeze until partially frozen, about 1 hour. Insert a stick in the center of each cup. Freeze until firm.

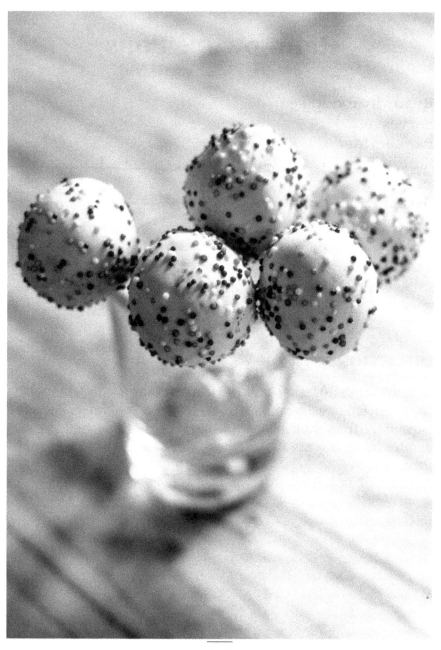

Vanilla Poached Peaches

Ready in about: 40 min
Serves: 4
Per serving:
Kcal 156, Sodium 2 mg, Protein 1 g, Carbs 38 g, Fat 3 g

INGREDIENTS:
- ½ cup sugar
- 1 cup of water
- 1 vanilla bean, split and scraped
- Mint leaves or cinnamon, for garnish
- 4 large peaches, pitted and quartered

DIRECTIONS:

Put the water, sugar, vanilla bean and scrapings in a saucepan. Mix the blend over a low heat until the sugar has dissolved. Continue to simmer until the mixture thickens, about 10 minutes. Add the sliced fruit. Cook over low heat for about 5 minutes. Transfer the peaches and sauce to small decorative bowls. Garnish with mint leaves or a pinch of cinnamon. Serve immediately.

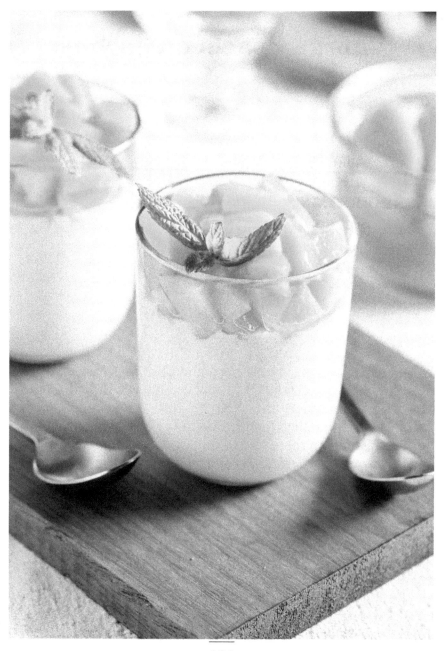

APPENDIX WITH CONVERSION CHARTS

WEIGHTS	
IMPERIAL	**METRIC**
½ oz.	15 g
¾ oz.	20 g
1 oz.	30 g
2 oz.	60 g
3 oz.	85 g
16 oz. = 1 pound= 435 g	
1 oz. = 28.35 g | 1 g = 0.035 oz.	

LIQUIDS

CUPS	METRIC	PINT	QUART
¼	60 ml	-	-
½	125 ml	-	-
-	150 ml	¼	-
-	200 ml	-	-
1	250 ml	½	-
-	300 ml	-	-
-	400 ml	-	-
2	500 ml	-	-
-	950 ml	-	1

SPOONS

LIQUID		DRY	
¼ tsp.	1.25 ml	¼ tsp.	1.1 g
½ tsp.	2.5 ml	½ tsp.	2.3 g
1 tsp.	5 ml	1 tsp.	4.7 g
¼ tbsp.	3.75 ml	¼ tbsp.	3.5 g
½ tbsp.	7.5 ml	½ tbsp.	7.1 g
1 tbsp.	15 ml	1 tbsp.	14.3 g

OVEN TEMPS

°F	°C
250	120
275	140
300	150
325	170
350	180
375	190
400	200

COMMON INGREDIENTS

1 CUP	IMPERIAL	METRIC
Flour	5 oz.	140 g
Almonds	4 oz.	110 g
Uncooked Rice	6½ oz.	190 g
Brown Sugar	6½ oz.	185 g
Raisins	7 oz.	200 g
Grated Cheese	4 oz.	115 g

NOTES

CPSIA information can be obtained
at www.ICGtesting.com
Printed in the USA
LVHW060953230421
685104LV00018B/176